MAGIC PLANTS

DE VEGETALIBUS MAGICIS

I0391056

First Edition 1700
M. Heucher

English Translation 1886
Edmund Goldsmid

New Edition 2016
Edited by Tarl Warwick

COPYRIGHT AND DISCLAIMER

FOREWORD

The following work is a compilation of two separate materials; a work by Heucher from the dawn of the 18th century on herbal magic, and some of the cults of old and their attempts to organize botanical materials according to the zodiac and in similar ways, twain with a sort of explanatory tract detailing several witch trials, probably to illustrate the dangers faced by then-modern rational individuals seeking to exonerate herbal healing from witchery in a more general sense.

The work is extremely dense; Heucher (translated by Goldsmid, who released several other private printings on spiritual topics around the same era) delves deeply into Egyptology and the Aesclepian system of the era, the concept of dreaming in order to obtain a cure or remedy, and such. Most interesting here is probably the observation that the number of, say, leaves or petals on a plant was used within numerically calculated magickal systems to denote the type of cure they represented, as well as their color in general relating to the same, or to the humors at large, or to constellations within astrological lore for medical purposes.

The witch trial material tacked onto the end is also of interest for here are two potentially herbal references also; one to witch ointment (now known to often be a tincture of belladonna, datura, henbane, or some combination of psychotropics) and the other to a mysterious black powder given to presumed witches by "The Devil" which caused disease or other problems to the victim.

This edition has been rendered into fully modern English. Care has been taken to retain all original intent and meaning.

INTRODUCTION

The curious tract translated in the following pages is one of those strange compositions written in the 17th century, wherein the writer, evidently a man of great erudition, endeavors to unmask what he considers the superstition of his age, but, in his attempt, at once exposes his own credulity.

The belief in Magic and Witchcraft was almost universal in the Middle Ages, and affected every class of Society, and all sorts and conditions of men. In our own country, as evidenced by our judicial records, the unreasoning credulity which swept across the civilized world, rose to high-water mark, assisted as it was by the efforts of that wise fool of a King, James the First of England and Sixth of Scotland.

Heucher's pamphlet itself is a small folio of 16 pp. I know of no copy besides my own, which formed part of the Maidment Library. The imprint is "Lipsiae, apud Paulum Ehrentium, MDCC." I have given, as an Appendix, a translation from the Official records of the Royal Court of Guernsey, of the trial of three women for witchcraft in 1617. This translation is taken from Mr. J. L. Pitt's Witchcraft and Devil-Lore in the Channel Islands. Anyone interested in the subject should get a copy of this very curious, interesting and really well edited pamphlet.

EDMUND GOLDSMID
Edinburgh, March 28th, 1886.

MAGIC PLANTS

Often and forcibly does it occur to me to wonder how it has happened that many men, of glorious reputation and famous for the greatness of their illustrious deeds, have believed in wicked and unlawful arts, yea, in some hidden compact entered upon with the devil. For, passing over the dreadful blasphemies of the Hebrew nation against the Savior, and the insolence of Hierocles accusing of sorcery both Him and his most holy disciples, chiefly Peter and Paul, and also the impious attacks of Plinius and Apuleius against Moses, and the false ideas of Theophilus of Alexandria and Eustathius of Antioch about Origen, and of the Arians about Athanasius; I find the great names of Pythagoras, Platinus, Jamblicus, Porphyrins, Chicus Aesculanus, Anselm of Parma, Peter of Aponum, Albertus Magnus, Frischlinus, Henricus Cornelius Agrippa, Michael Scott, and Roger Bacon, and finally the names of even the Popes Sylvester II. and Gregory VII. mentioned in the catalogs of renowned Magicians.

And concerning all of these, it is clearly confirmed that they stood out from the crowd as illustrious and of great celebrity, as men whom a lofty spirit and intellect separated from the vulgar herd of literati; a careful study of astrology and nature gave them an understanding of all the most abstruse questions, and transmitted their brilliant theories even to posterity, so that it seems to be almost superfluous for any one, after the example of Gabriel Naudaeus, to defend them by a written apology. But I ceased to wonder when I thought of envy, the assiduous companion of virtue, and when I noticed how much it prevails, nay, even when I considered the grounds that may have led to such belief. There are such very wicked examples of profane deceivers meeting us in every age, that I need not go into ancient history, sacred or profane ; the more recent writings of Doctor

5

MAGIC PLANTS

Faust, Zedechias the Jew, Scotus Parvus, Christopherus Wageners, the three Eschelles, of Merlinus and Maugis, or of Naudaeus (if you prefer magic romances) suffice. Their tricks and manifold deceits, although not to be compared with the wonderful works of wisdom and art carried out by the learned men mentioned before, made a deep impression, however, owing to the particularly gross ignorance of the ages in which they lived, but they also left on them an indelible blot of infamy.

For such barbarity and want of knowledge existed in their time, that every class of learning which was not of the common kind was looked upon with suspicion, and men, carried away by their own base ideas, erroneously thought it had been drawn from the most filthy lake of hell. And, indeed, a more just or more accurate judgment could scarcely be expected from those men, since, besides their utter ignorance of literature, they were also ignorant of real magic, which embraces in its sphere the highest culminating point of all sciences, and by the help of which rare, abstruse, and unaccustomed effects are produced.

For, be it far from me to assent to the opinion of those who, with Thomas Erastus and his defender Georgius Hornius, renounce all magic and condemn it as illicit and low; since all those reasons which they have hitherto brought before the public are open to many objections, and if they do prove anything, it is nothing else than that the legitimate use of magic, as very often happens in other cases, has been brought into disrepute by abuse. People in general are hardly cautious enough, and are a little too violent and abusive regarding lawful magic, looking upon it as being unlawful and being accustomed to call it forbidden, devilish, deceitful, supernatural, poisonous, black, foul, base, of had repute, the evil art and other names.

These men indeed, believe as Democritus, Averhoes, and

MAGIC PLANTS

Simplicius do, that there are no devils. They either attribute all results to good angels, whom by reason of their superiority they call spirits, and argue that our air is full of them; to which class belong the Platonics, Jamblicus, Porphyrius, Proclus and Julian the Emperor; or else they think, with Avicenna and Petrus Pomponatius his pupil, that all things spring from hidden magnetic properties, and a peculiar state of the atmosphere, or with Reginald Scott trace back most cases to madness, black bile, or other disturbances of nature, or along with Thomas Campanella, and Marcus Marx, believe in the power of concentrated will. I may mention Cornelius Loosens, Gallidus Gaudanus, Robertus Fludd, John Weir, Bodinus, and many others as supporting my contention, since it can be seen by their writings that they believed in such a thing as beneficent sorcery.

Therefore, both these opinions being considered, it may be as well to conclude that magic is not altogether to be renounced and despised, since some magic may be found, which is not only free from wickedness, but which even deserves much commendation. Although I would willingly grant that what is base and devilish, is often blended with that blameless and harmless science, just as that science in an impure state often advances in the guise of one which is legitimate, and adopts methods from nature. This the most ancient of the Magi had already done, as Lucanus, Statius, Seneca the tragedian, and others assert. For they wished to appear to have accomplished every thing they did by the power of Nature. Whence you often read that they invoked Hecate, since by her they specified nature herself, or the Empress of Nature, which fact the passage in Eusebius, in Prapar. Evatzg. makes tolerably clear, wherein Hecate says of herself : "Bearing the threefold symbols of a threefold nature."

Nay, what hinders me from stating with Vossius *de Orig. et Pror. Idol.*, that evil spirits accomplish nothing save by natural powers, and that nothing can be done except by the powers of nature. For what, pray, if the power they have of moving themselves and other bodies separate from them, of driving forward or backward the elements, of transporting weights as if by machinery, of gathering things scattered and scattering things gathered, of hiding things seen, of assuming other bodies, of applying actives to passives, of changing organism itself, of destroying sensations, and of accomplishing innumerable other things; what is all this whereby they strive to deceive men, but making use of of natural forces?

All these things have such a considerable bearing on our theme, that they are altogether worthy of being duly inquired into. There are many effects which we see produced, particularly admirable and unusual, which must be attributed to the Supreme Deity alone, and on that account you may consistently call them supernatural, since by a long distance they outstrip the usual powers of nature. Others indeed, springing from the same Creator, owe nevertheless their whole beginning to the motion, imparted and definitely implanted by fixed laws in the system of the world at its creation, and are therefore simply called natural.

Others indeed, differ from these to this extent, that they depend chiefly on our imagination, the stupendous power of which let us not treat too lightly. And we believe there are some allied to these, which emanate from superstition, as Theophastus very well shows in his Characters.

Finally, certain results which we are able to assign to none of these classes of causes yet enumerated, are attributed to the devil, and thus belong to the supernatural. Being so far removed from God, they have been distinguished by the name of devilish. Moreover, to this list I would add all those, which although they depend on, and proceed solely from, some evident natural cause, nevertheless, because the devil mixes himself up with them, pretends that they are his own work and feigns that he is their author, deserve to be called devilish as well as magical.

For, indeed, what powerful mind is not able to perceive by fair investigation, how feebly, how confusedly, and with what small degree of accuracy, these subjects are handled in the writings of most men, for, although we have a very bountiful supply of authors on this theme, so much so that, if you wished to estimate the number of those who have written on magic, your paper would hardly contain them, you will nevertheless be unable to name one who has unfolded and explained everything, as was befitting. I will not, at this time, discuss all magic, which indeed, these little pages would not contain, but I place before myself, as my theme, for the present at least, the vegetable kingdom alone, in which, the industry, if not of all, at any rate of many has failed to enlighten us, and since, so far as I know, former writers have recorded in their writings far too little about magical plants, I will devote myself to this, if I may use the expression, fruitful subject. Poets (since frequent mention of the subject is made in their writings,) must have been aware that thereafter, its usefulness would be fully appreciated. For, who can forget the powerful and noxious herbs of Medea, the enchanting herbs of Lucan, the fatal herbs of Claudian, the flourishing plants of Maro, and lastly those venomous plants, of which abundance was to be found in Colchis and Thessally?

Who is ignorant of the Nepenthe of Homer, the Polion of Hesiod, the plant of the Ethiopians drying up waters, the Asphodel, sweet food of the Manes, the plant of Juba and Bela arousing the dead, the soothsaying The langis, the Juniper and Hypericum putting the demons to flight, the Alyssus, Baccharis, Adianthus, Satyrion and the Amulets of the Syderii charms against witchcraft?

Nevertheless it has not yet appeared necessary to any

one to explain these mysteries so that the observant reader might rest satisfied with regard to them. Which fact therefore the more impels me to embrace the opportunity.

I confess that, at first, I was filled with no inconsiderable joy when I read the list of the authors who have spoken of magic, not without praise- Hermes, Orpheus, Museeus, Pythagoras, Democritus, Empedocles, Kiranus, and others, all of whom are said to have praised magical plants; from this I promised myself a great solace to my labor. But, indeed, all hope immediately came to naught when I found that most of these authors had been destroyed by the injury of time, or if any fragments of their writings survive they are of uncertain and slight reliance, as there is still much doubt as to the real authorship of such fragments.

Nor do the writers whose works on plants survive satisfy my expectations much more- namely, Theophrastus Eresius, Plinius, Apuleius, and those who have drawn small streams from these sources- Theophrastus, Paracelsus, Th. Cantipratanus, the feigned name of Albert the Great, Bernh. G. Penotus, Alex. Suchtenius, Leonh. Turnheuserus, Carrichterus, Mich. Sendigovius, Jo. Ern. Burggravius, Wreckerus, Porta, Lemnius, and a few others. These writers on plants, on the wonders of nature and other hidden things, however much they may wish to appear to have founded the healing effects of herbs on natural laws, either wittingly or corrupted by superstition, have nevertheless inserted in their writings certain things which savor somewhat of magic and supernatural agency.

It behooves the mind to approach this subject free from every preconceived notion and superstition, and properly imbued with natural science and learning, nay, even with a knowledge of the healing art itself. For when those who first wrote on the subject gave their attention almost solely to meditation about the stars, and believed natural philosophy and the healing art to be intimately connected with these heavenly bodies, they disseminated seeds of magic, from which that science grew to such a degree that it overspread the whole world with its pollution. Of this fact Pliny is a remarkable witness in his Natural History, confirming what we have said by these words:

"No one can doubt that magic is the greatest of the sciences, seeing that it is the only one which embraces three other sciences having power over the human mind, and reduces them to one. No one doubts that it has sprung from medicine, and become something loftier and holier than its parent."

This is what Grillus also maintains, saying that all the Egyptians are physicians. From which fact it is clearly proved that the healing art almost always flourished among that nation, and thus, as we shall soon show, contributed much to our argument.

I will not flatter myself that this work will be so complete as to appear perfect in all parts before the learned world. It is sufficient to have wished to make it so, in so far as it goes. I have written this present work on the so-called vegetable kingdom, including and embracing in its limits nothing less than all that springs from the soil, and is thus brought into existence, to germinate, be nourished and increase, both in roots, leaves, stalks, stems, flowers, branches, twigs, fruits and seeds. In short, nothing in this work belongs either to the animal or mineral kingdoms, and let it be remembered that magic specifies not merely what is devilish, but also all that which is considered supernatural through ignorance and superstition.

Since therefore, I intend to treat of magical herbs, I will specially enumerate if not all, at least most plants, herbs, trees, leaves, flowers, fruits and seeds, which are considered to savor of anything superstitious and deceitful, and those by means of which the great author of falsehoods imposes on men; and then, as far as I can, I will inquire into the causes of the effects attributed to these herbs.

And, from this little work of mine, I hope not only that some advantage will accrue to those who long to understand many of the more obscure passages of old authors, but I also believe that many of the deceptions practiced by sorcerers will be detected, by which it is possible that our knowledge of natural philosophy, as well as of medicine may greatly be increased.

Wherefore, if any one is resolved to commence from the beginning, he, in my opinion, will not be far wrong if, first of all, he seek the origin of science in the study of old authors on the healing art. Thus, although the first principles of the science ought rightly and deservedly to be attributed to the Egyptians-whose very ancient records, however, are far from clear- yet these elements are by no means free from superstition, for Africa is considered the mother of all unnatural things. Different, indeed, was the reasoning of the Egyptians from that of Aristotle.

For he, dealing with the interpretation of dreams, decided that no dreams were sent by the Gods to men, as it was unworthy of their dignity to go into the couches of sleepers and disturb the weary. The Egyptians, on the contrary, when they were about to consult destiny regarding the cure of any severe and particularly desperate disease, having duly purified their mind before they betook themselves to the couch, used to wait for the revelations of the Gods in their dreams, and according to the dictates of these revelations, used this or that method of cure.

As this rite was a little too simple at first, so in process of time, it was more and more overloaded with ceremonies. For, when many plants and flowers had come under the notice of the sorcerers, they, with the selfish imagination of enthusiasts grew to consider them as favors stored up beforehand for themselves. Then they besought heaven and the Gods with hymns, to show by means of a dream, which plants were the best cure for the disease, then, after preparing themselves by prayer to sleep, whatever deity first appeared to them in their dream was supposed to indicate the plant specially attributed to him, as the one divinely destined to subdue the disease. Which fact Jamblicus, referring to the Egyptian mysteries, testifies to in the following words: "Thus, in the temple of Aesculapius, diseases are cured by divine dreams, and the healing art arose from holy dreams," And Aristides further confirms this.

Not that the Egyptians, at the shrines of Isis, Osiris, and of the Egyptian Aesculapius, which was close by the banks of the Nile, followed this custom in the same manner as the Greeks and Romans in the temples of Hephestion or Vulcan, but the general process was as familiar to the Greeks and Romans as to the Egyptians. For, with this intention and design, the former often used to sleep in the temple of Aesculapius, to which custom Aristophanes refers when he says:

"Let both you and I go as soon as possible, and lie down in the temple of Aesculapius." Which rite Plautus also alluded to in Latin; "Therefore it happens that this sick procurer lies in the temple of Aesculapius." They were accustomed to act in the same way in this temple, as in the city of Pergamos in Asia, whither Herodianus states that Antoninus Caracalla had set out, "wishing to use the cures of Aesculapius." The same thing used to take place in the temple of the Oropian Amphiarus, about which Pausanias says: "Sacrificing a ram to him, and spreading out the skin to sleep, waiting for the appearance of the dream."

And from these testimonies of authors it is pretty clear, how remarkably the "lying down" of the Greeks, and the zealously "watching the gods" of the Latins, the hides of those, and the couches of these, corresponded to one another, all of which things have reference to the custom of sleeping in temples and to the rite of lying in wait for divine revelations to be obtained by means of sleep. In very truth, what class of vulgar dreams these were, those may judge, who know how perverse and idolatrous a worship of the gods prevailed in those times, and what sort of deities the heathen worshiped and honored. I, indeed, have no doubt that the devil was by no means forgetful of himself, but was chiefly intent on his own profit, and that he had embraced this suitable and very convenient opportunity of defiling the natural and healing Science by means of the most wicked superstitions. Which thing even Borrichius in other passages the keenest opponent of Couringuis, who thinks along with us, considers necessary to confess in his book on the hermetic art, and on account of this, thinks that we should lament the miseries of these nations estranged from the true worship of the deity.

Nevertheless, Kircherus in his Oedipus Aegyptiacus, seems to have spoken too strongly about these enchantments of dreamers, since he thought that, although this plan of curing afforded wonderful results even in lamentable diseases, these were by no means to be ascribed to the natural power and quality of the plants, but to a hidden compact and treaty with demons.

For although very often cures have been effected, the plants used in which have been only an outward sign, the devils supplying the actual power of curing, no one, nevertheless, will hesitate to assert that none of those remedies, acting in a natural way, have displayed a power and efficacy of their own.

And so the Egyptians obtained some fair knowledge of plants, and did not remain content with dreams, but advanced even further. They had, indeed, selected from those who had appeared to the dreamers ten gods, whom they used especially to entreat to show the readiest cures of diseases. To each of these they had given a separate number- number one to the Supreme Deity and the Cause of Causes, number two to Mephta, number three to Minerva, number four to Apollo or Horus, number five to Isis, number six to Osiris, number seven to Mercury, number eight to Ammon, number nine to Typhon, lastly, number ten to Momphta, and they had thus come to connect numbers with the gods. Thereafter they examined the numbers the leaves, plants, and flowers had, how many pips fruit contained, and how many joints stems possessed, and afterwards considered them sacred to that god whose number was thus represented, and placed them under his guardianship. Nor did they attend to the number only, but earnestly watched the color and the form in flowers; and as regards stalks of plants, they duly inquired whether they were round, smooth, three-sided or four-sided, and dedicated these stalks as scepters to the corresponding deities, as can be further proved from the Bembina Fabula in the writings of Kircherus.

They used to believe that they were able to show wonderful results, which fact the sublime Platonic Proclus, in his book concerning sacrifices and magic, besides others, confirms. He adds that by amalgamation of many things they obtained supernatural influence, but he thinks, nevertheless, that sometimes one plant or one stone has been sufficient for the divine work, adding that in stones and plants is concentrated the essence of divine powers.

Further, the chemical plants, which (if we believe Origen and Stobseus) were thirty-six in number, clearly prove this very thing. For, dividing the whole human body into so many parts, they assigned a separate divinity to each, whether god or devil; or, with Galenus and J. M. Firmicus, you may call them decani; each of whom was the presiding genius who looked after the safety of his own appointed limb or member.

MAGIC PLANTS

And if a man lost the health of any member they persuaded themselves that it could be recovered, its respective deity being invoked by the name peculiar to himself, and propitiated by the plant dedicated to himself. Firmicus, Haephestion the Theban, and Manlius differ among themselves about the Decani and their number, whether there were thirty-six only, three always being given to each sign of the zodiac, or whether, indeed, there were more; or whether every one of these had under him his own subordinates and fellow workers. I am content to believe that they were divided according to the twelve signs of the zodiac, possessed of unlimited power over the whole human body, and were wont to be propitiated by certain plants.

Nay, it was a proper and extremely common custom to appoint to separate signs- nay, to separate constellations- their own herbs; Abenrahman, the Arabian philosopher, moreover, relates that they chose for use as medicines all forms of nature and grades of beings which possessed any resemblance to, or quality in common with, the seven planets. As an example, all forms which bore any resemblance to the sun they chose from minerals, metals, stones, animals, plants, and herbs, and turned them to use as medicine for the heart, because the heart is, as it were, the sun of a smaller world; which things can be still more comprehensively read in Jamblichus's De Mysteriis Aegyptiortun, Marsilius, and likewise in Ficinus.

Who does not see that later, further superstitions sprang from this connection of plants with Heavenly bodies, and among these I may specially mention the belief that the efficacy of the plants depended on the hour they were gathered in the meadows, which hour was fixed by the influence of the stars.

And those will not oppose this base and false custom, who still believe that greater powers lie in the stems of Hypericum, dug up on the Feast of St. John, in twigs of the wild cherry cut off on the sacred anniversary of St. Martin, and in the sympathetic ashen wood, split up at noon, when the sun is in the sign Virgo, and the moon in a crescent state. Of this superstition Keinsius (in var. lect. Freitag. noct. med.), Maxwellus (Medicin. Magnet.) and Grabius, (Arcan. Medic.) supply many examples. Kircherus tries to prove that, particularly at the time of the solstice, the leaves of the willow, white poplar, elm, lime, and olive turn their underside to the sky; for this very reason, therefore, I am not willing to leave out of account all motions of the heavenly bodies; besides, in the work of Gesnerus, we come across not a few examples of plants having been affected in shape by the sun and moon, this being a clear proof of harmony with their own constellations.

Much less do I strive to reject or reproach all plucking of plants at fixed times as being an unnecessary process, desiring merely to prove, with Couringius, that the idea of the risings, settings, and positions of the constellations fixing the different times of collection, is ridiculous, and moreover, that the belief that we can determine the very days, hours, and even minutes, savors altogether of superstition, and by no means differs from the doctrines of the Egyptians. Which ideas Helmontius refutes uncommonly well, and censures in the following words. He says:

"In modern books on Medicine there be some who ascribes a great number of diseases to signs of the Zodiac, and since the number of these signs was too small, they extended each into three sections, in order, forsooth, to divide all herbs into thirty six classes. Do we not know that the soil has a capacity of raising plants from itself, which capacity, therefore, it need not beg from heaven."

Finally, concerning the apportionment of plants to the seven planets I have nothing to say, except that the very number of the planets now known sufficiently silences the theory.

MAGIC PLANTS

Neither, however, is it right, in making researches about plants, to believe that all the science of the Egyptians was magic; although I cannot but greatly approve of the way they judged of the excellence of herbs by the help of their external senses. Nay, even he may not have erred who has said that these men surpassed in many ways the carefulness of later writers, when, besides taste and smell, which almost alone you see our botanists employ, they also summoned to their assistance hearing, sight, and touch. With the help of the ear they judged by the sharp, heavy, ringing, dull, harsh, or gentle sound, of the consistency of the stem; by the hand, from the smoothness, roughness, softness, or hardness, of its texture; and lastly, by the eyes they decided from the colors as to the virtues lurking within.

Thus, by judging carefully from their senses, they were able to infer and learn the effects of plants.

But, truly, the more correctly they conducted themselves in this matter the more basely did they devote themselves to superstition. Carefully they used to watch for the distinctive mark of every plant, observed to which member of the human body it corresponded, and carefully noted the result, afterwards thinking that plant most suitable to that limb which it resembled by its own external shape. Or by a certain supposed analogy of qualities, they applied it as a remedy to that limb. Thus the peony flowers yet enclosed in the bud and poppy heads they dedicated to the head. In like manner the Euphrastia, Caltha, Heiracius, and Anthemis they thought beneficial to the eyes, because in them they found something of the first elements of the eye; they assigned the root of the Dentaria to the teeth, of the Anthora to the heart. If, therefore, they came across any plant, the Cynosorchis, for example, like the genitals in shape, they persuaded themselves that it most certainly cured the sexual passions, since by its influence they believed that deity could be summoned who presided over the genitals.

MAGIC PLANTS

For a like reason, also, they employed the juices of plants which in color resembled the juices or humors of the human body, for the purpose of cleansing it of the offending humor. Hence, they wished to cure the yellow bile with the saffron colored juices of plants, the black bile with the black, purple or azure phlegm with the white, blood with the red, and milk and semen with (he juices resembling milk. Whence it can be inferred that this science was not, as many (among whom is Couringius) think, invented in modern times, but that it was raised afresh from the records of Eastern people, since very distinct proofs of this are found in the writings of Dioscoris and Pliny, and, probably, from the absurd customs of the Egyptians. I confess that, on this point, I rather prefer now to suspend my judgment than to settle on anything as certain. For even if the opponents of this theory maintain that it follows as a consequence from it that the fruit of the Anacardium, for example, must be the best cordial, that the famous Cephalic must produce the best apples; the Aphrodisiac, the best plums; and the juice of the Esula the best milk; they nevertheless prove nothing from that, as it can be at once retorted: How long is it since Mercury, Antimony, Cinnabar, Coriander seeds, etc, were excluded from the list of poisons? Borriclius argues as follows:

"It is a characteristic of human, not of Divine nature, to inquire remissly into things. Nothing has ever been discovered or created until after many weak and apparently futile efforts."

Those are the original fibers, as it were, from which the tree of the belief in the magic virtues of plants grew to such an extent, as to spread its branches so widely that it refuses to be embraced in these narrow limits. It is a matter of inquiry even whether the land of the Egyptians supplied itself with its own magic plants. Couringius shows that it furnished a few wines, but did not abound in medicinal remedies. Let writers contend among themselves as long as they wish, we refer those who desire to know more to the books on Egyptian plants published by Kircher and other writers, from which each can form his own opinion. But now, I regret that I am prevented by the limits of my parchment from entering into any disquisition concerning the merits of these plants, whose names I have recorded.

There are indeed among their number some of such a nature, that I may briefly mention their names and properties: the Salvia, Veratrum, Juniperus, etc, powerful in routing the demons; the Adianthus, Ruta, Sideritis, etc, a sovereign charm for overcoming witchcraft; the Absinthium, Ricinus, Cnebison, Scordotis, etc, used in sacrifices, and to obtain divine apparitions; the Asphodel, irresistible in calling forth the gloomy deities and the Manes; the Osiris, etc, which enables one to prophesy; the Laurus, Theangelis, Halicaccabi, Bellonasia, Vatica, etc, which bring on madness, ravings and sleep; Strichnon, Thallassegle, Gelotophyllis, Semasum, the plant of Nectanebus, the Olive, Mandragora, Catanance, Cemos, Anacampserotis, etc, which enter into the composition of aphrodisiacs or love-potions. The Pleiracium, Theombrotium, Bali, Juba, etc, said to have power to rouse from death itself. I shall with care explain, time and opportunity permitting, the qualities of these and many other plants, but meanwhile I must bid thee farewell, benevolent reader.

END OF MAGIC PLANTS

APPENDIX

CONFESSIONS OF WITCHES UNDER TORTURE

Before Amice De Carteret, Esq., Bailiff, and the Jurats.
July 4th, 1617.

Sentence of Death.

Collette du Mont, widow of Jean Becquet; Marie, her daughter, wife of Pierre Massy; and Isabel Becquet, wife of Jean Le Moygne, being by common rumor and report for a long time past addicted to the damnable art of Witchcraft, and the same being thereupon seized and apprehended by the Officers of His Majesty (James I.), after voluntarily submitting themselves, both upon the general inquest of the country, and after having been several times brought up before the Court, heard, examined, and confronted, upon a great number of depositions made and produced before the Court by the said Officers; from which it is clear and evident that for many years past the aforesaid women have practiced the diabolical art of Witchcraft, by having not only cast their spells upon inanimate objects, but also by having retained in languor through strange diseases, many persons and beasts; and also cruelly hurt a great number of men, women, and children, and caused the death of many animals, as recorded in the informations thereupon laid, it follows that they are clearly convicted and proved to be Witches. In expiation of which crime it has been ordered by the Court that the said women shall be presently conducted, with halters about their necks, to the usual place of punishment, and shall there be fastened by the Executioner to a gallows, and be hanged, strangled, killed, and burnt, until their flesh and bones are reduced to ashes, and the ashes shall be scattered; and all their goods, chattels, and estates, if any such exist, shall be forfeited to His Majesty. In order to make them disclose their accomplices, they shall be put to the question before the Court, previous to being executed.

Sentence of Death having been pronounced against Collette Du Mont, widow of Jean Becquet; Marie, her daughter, wife of Pierre Massy; and Isabel Becquet, wife of Jean Le Moygne; the same have confessed as follows:

CONFESSION OF COLLETTE DU MONT

First, the said Collette immediately after the said sentence was pronounced, and before leaving the Court, freely admitted that she was a Witch at the same time, not wishing to specify the crimes which she had committed, she was taken, along with the others, to the Torture Chamber, and the said question being applied to her, she confessed that she was quite young when the Devil, in the form of a cat* appeared to her; in the Parish of Torteval, as she was returning from her cattle, it being still daylight, and that he took occasion to lead her astray by inciting her to avenge herself on one of her neighbors, with whom she was then at enmity, on account of some damage which she had suffered through the cattle of the latter; that since then when she had a quarrel with anyone, he appeared to her in the aforesaid form, and sometimes-

*As regards these colons, occurring where they are not required, Mr Pitts observes that they correspond to similar pauses in the original records, and evidently indicate the successive stages by which the story was wrung from the wretched victims. They are thus endowed with a sad and ghastly significance, for it must be remembered that the confessions were not made in a connected form, but were elicited by leading questions, often accompanied by a fresh spell of torture.

-in the form of a dog : inducing her to take vengeance upon those who had angered her, persuading her to cause the death of persons and cattle. That the Devil having come to fetch her that she might go to the Sabbath, called for her without anyone perceiving it, and gave her a certain black ointment with which (after having stripped herself), she rubbed her back, belly and stomach, and then having again put on her clothes, she went out of her door, when she was immediately carried through the air at a great speed, and she found herself in an instant at the place of the Sabbath, which was sometimes near the parochial burial-ground, and at other times near the seashore in the neighborhood of Rocquaine Castle, where, upon arrival, she met often fifteen or sixteen Wizards and Witches with the Devils who were there in the form of dogs, cats, and hares, which Wizards and Witches she was unable to recognize, because they were all blackened and disfigured, it was true, however, that she had heard the Devil summon them by their names, and she remembered among others those of Fallaise and Hardie, confessed that on entering the Sabbath, the Devil wishing to summon them commenced with her sometimes. Admitted that her daughter Marie, wife of Massy, now condemned for a similar crime, was a Witch, and that she took her twice to the Sabbath with her, at the Sabbath, after having worshiped the Devil, who used to stand up on his hind legs, they had connection with him under the form of a dog, then they danced back to back. And after having danced, they drank wine (she did not know what color it was), which the Devil poured out of a jug into a silver or pewter goblet, which wine did not seem to her so good as that which was usually drunk; they also ate white bread which he presented to the- she had never seen any salt at the Sabbath.

Confessed that the Devil had charged her to call, as she passed, for Isabel le Moygne, when she came to the Sabbath, which she had done several times. On leaving the Sabbath the Devil incited her to commit various evil deeds, and to that effect he gave her certain black powders, which he ordered her to throw upon such persons and cattle as she wished; with this powder she perpetrated several wicked acts which she did not remember, among others she threw some upon Mr Dolbell, parish minister, and was the occasion of his death by these means. With this same powder she bewitched the wife of Jean Maugues, but denied that the woman's death was caused by it, she also touched on the side, and threw some of this powder over the deceased wife of Mr Perchard, the minister who succeeded the said Dolbell in the parish, she being enceinte at the time, and so caused the death of her and her infant- she did not know that the deceased woman had given her any cause for doing so.

Upon the refusal of the wife of Collas Totte-vin to give her some milk, she caused her cow to dry up, by throwing upon it some of this powder; which cow she afterwards cured again by making it eat some bran, and some terrestrial herb that the Devil gave her.

CONFESSION OF MARIE BECQUET

Marie, wife of Pierre Massy, after sentence of death had been pronounced against her, having been put to the question, confessed that she was a Witch; and that at the persuasion of the Devil, who appeared to her in the form of a dog; she gave herself to him, that when she gave herself to him he took her by the hand with his paw, that she used to anoint herself with the same ointment as her mother used, and had been to the Sabbath upon the bank near Rocquaine Castle with her, where there was no one but the Devil and her as it seemed, in the aforesaid form in which she had seen him several times. She was also at the Sabbath on one occasion among others in the road near Collas Tottevin's; every time that she went to the Sabbath, the Devil came to her, and it seemed as though he transformed her into a female dog; she said that upon the shore, near the said

Rocquaine. The Devil, in the form of a dog, having had connection with her, gave her bread and wine, which she ate and drank.

The Devil gave her certain powders; which powders he put into her hand, for her to throw upon those whom he ordered her, she threw some of them by his orders upon persons and cattle; notably upon the child of Pierre Brehaut. Item, upon the wife of Jean Bourgatze, while she was enceinte. Item, upon the child of Leonard le Messurier.

CONFESSION OF ISABEL BECQUET

Isabel, wife of Jean le Moygne, having been put to the question, at once confessed that she was a Witch; and that upon her getting into a quarrel with the woman Girarde, who was her sister-in-law; the Devil, in the form of a hare, took occasion to tempt her; appearing to her in broad daylight in a road near her house, and persuading and inciting her to give herself to him, and that he would help her to avenge herself on the said Girarde, and everybody else, to which persuasion she would not at the moment condescend to yield, so he at once disappeared, but very soon he came again to her in the same road, and pursuing his previous argument, exhorted her in the same terms as above, that done, he left her and went away, after having previously given her a sackful of parsnips, she then took a certain black powder wrapped in a cloth in which he placed it, which powder she kept by her. He appeared to her another time under the same form in the town district, inciting her anew to give herself to him, but she not wishing to comply, he next made a request to her to give him some living animal; whereupon she returned to her dwelling and fetched a chicken which she carried to him to the same place where she had left him, and he took it, and after having thanked her he made an appointment for her to be present the next morning before daylight at the Sabbath, promising that he would send for her according to which promise, during the ensuing night, the old woman Collette du Mont, came to fetch her, and gave her some black ointment, which she had had from the Devil; with this (after having stripped herself) she anointed her back and belly, then having dressed herself again she went out of her house door, when she was instantly caught up, and carried across hedges and bushes to the bank on the sea shore, in the neighborhood of Rocquaine Castle, the usual place where the Devil kept his Sabbath. No sooner had she arrived there than the Devil came to her in the form of a dog, with two great horns sticking up; and with one of his paws (which seemed to her like hands) took her by the hand, and calling her by her name told her that she was welcome, then immediately the Devil made her kneel down, while he himself stood up on his hind legs; he then made her express detestation of the Eternal in these words: I renounce God the Father, God the Son, and God the Holy Ghost . And then caused her to worship and invoke himself in these terms; Our Great Master, help us! with a special compact to be faithful to him, and when this was done he had connection with her in the aforesaid form of a dog, but a little larger, then she and the others danced with him back to back: After having danced, the Devil poured out of a jug some black wine, which he presented to them in a wooden bowl, from which she drank, but it did not seem to her so good as the wine which is usually drunk: There was also bread but she did not eat any, confessed that she gave herself to him for a month; they returned from the Sabbath in the same manner that they went there.

The second time she was at the Sabbath was after the old woman Collette had been to fetch her, and she anointed herself with the ointment as above stated; declared, that on entering the Sabbath, she again had connection with the Devil and danced with him; after having danced, and upon his solicitation to prolong the time, she gave herself to him for three years; at the Sabbath the Devil used to summon the Wizards and Witches in regular order (she remembered very well having heard him call the old woman Collette the first, in these terms: Madame the Old Woman Becquette), then the woman Fallane, and afterwards the woman Hardie. Item, he also called Marie, wife of Massy, and daughter of the said Collette. Said that after them she herself was called by the Devil, in these terms, The Little Becquette: she also heard him call there Collas Becquet, son of the said old woman (who (Collas) held her by the hand in dancing, and someone (a woman) whom she did not know, held her by the other hand). There were about six others there she did not know; the said old woman was always nearest to the Devil, occasionally while some were dancing, others were having connection with the Devils in the form of dogs. They remained at the Sabbath about three or four hours, not more. While at the Sabbath the Devil marked her at the upper part of the thigh, which mark having been examined by the midwives, they reported that they had stuck a small pin deeply into it, and that she had not felt it, and that no blood had issued; she did not know in what part the Devil had marked the others, those who came first to the place of the Sabbath, waited for the others, and all the Wizards and Witches appeared in their proper forms; but blackened and disfigured so that they could not be recognized.

The Devil appeared sometimes in the form of a goat at the Sabbath; never saw him in other forms, on their departure he made them kiss him behind, and asked them when they would come again, he exhorted them always to be true to him, and to do evil deeds, and to this end he gave them certain black powders, wrapped in a cloth, for them to throw upon those whom they wished to bewitch. On leaving the Sabbath, the Devil went away in one direction and they in the other, after he had taken them all by the hand. At the instigation of the Devil she threw some of the powder over several persons and cattle; notably over Jean Jehan, when he came to her house to look for a pig. Item, over the child of James Gallienne, and over others. Item, over the cattle of

Brouart, and of others.

It was the Devil that was seen at the said Gallienne's house in the form of a rat and a weasel, she herself being then in the neighborhood of Gallienne's house, and he (the Devil) came to her in the form of a man, and struck her several blows on the face and head, by which she was bruised and torn in the way that she was seen the next day by Thomas Sohier, And she believed that the cause of this maltreatment was because she would not go with the Devil to the house of the said Gallienne.

She never went to the Sabbath except when her husband remained all night fishing at sea.

Whenever she wanted to bewitch anyone and her powder happened to have been all used up, the Devil appeared to her and told her to go to such a place, which he named, for some more, and when she did so, she never failed to find it there.

THE END

www.ingramcontent.com/pod-product-compliance
Lightning Source LLC
Chambersburg PA
CBHW061454180526
45170CB00004B/1697